BLOOMING FROM YOUR ASHES

A SPECIAL THANK YOU:

There are many Leaders and Spiritual Messengers who have fed me all the way from childhood to now. We don't learn on our own, we learn from reading, from listening and being open-minded to growth and by expanding our contribution to this existence over time. We learn from who we surround ourselves with, whether in person, on social media, or who we watch/listen to speak. We learn and we grow when we make the decision to utilize our hardships and love harder, rather than becoming hard and cold. None of this is mine, it is theirs-and now it is yours to share. Every single soul who has taught me, through love and lessons, heartache and loss, victories and defeats, I am eternally grateful for who I've had the pleasure of loving while I've been here. This is my Pay-It-Forward Message of Hope.

Thank you to those who have taught me, and to those who I pray continue to learn from me.

Thank you to my Lyla Girl for being my daily mirror of the God in me.

INTRODUCTION

You could be at any point in your life in picking this book up, but regardless of how you're *feeling* at this current stage of your being, it isn't coincidence that you're reading these words. Maybe you're one of the blessed souls that is on the brink of achieving your dreams as we speak, or maybe you're in a state of complacency and going through the motions of what the world wants of you each day; maybe you're in a place of deep sadness or sorrow. Regardless of where you are in your path, if you choose to read these words with an open mind, you could be giving yourself the opportunity to change *everything* for yourself - all on your own, **for good.**

Whether you've ever really known yourself or your direction, or you're just now at a point in your journey of wanting to dig a little deeper and know the value of your life beyond your past experiences and daily struggles, my hope is that this will add a great dose of hope and clarity to your life.

If you do not make a choice about how this life will be lived, your life will inevitably make the choice for you.

If you're feeling a bit lost, you're not as far off as you feel you may be. The simple action of you opening the cover of this book out of curious hope, means that you are craving more of *something* out of this existence, and *that...that* is what I am here to present to you: More from the life that you are currently living-no matter where you are at in your story.

This is a collection of some of the real-life lessons and encounters that I have learned from walking my path, that have taught me how to more than just merely survive each day and go through the motions, but how to thrive in my soul and crave *more* every single day. I have many Spiritual and Life Leaders who have contributed to the lessons in which I want to teach to you. I want to share with you some of what I have learned, in hopes that you will spend a whole lot less time putting yourself through as much hell as I did, once you have heard some truths that resonate with you.

A few truths to begin:

-You were not meant to roam this existence in a "living death," going through the motions without a direction all your own.

-You were not built or created to just be here and have the world show you where you belong.

-Life is not meant to feel constantly heavy.

-No matter which religion or background you wear, it isn't meant to keep you from a life of love and light and freedom of peace.

-You were born enough.

-All on your own.

-You were born powerful and capable and with this rare, individual greatness inside of you that nobody in this existence could ever steal, replace or duplicate, no matter how hard they try. Deep down, you **know** that already.

You were just also born into, raised or taught over time in surroundings that may have been very different than you, and it has taught and convinced you that you must stay there, and *there* is not where you belong.

You deserve to live in a place in your soul that is so confident, joyous, peaceful and loving that the world outside of you doesn't have a choice but to adapt to your level of being, rather than it changing what is within you.

I am not here to tell you what to do or how to live your life, I am here to tell you that *you* deserve the life you have always dreamed - the relationships that you have been so desperate to seek, and the peace and contentment you crave so deeply.

You deserve a shot at being the *BEST* version of yourself before you make the decision to give up.

If who you are today doesn't want to be here and doesn't care what happens to you one way or the other; if who you are today is checked out and hurt and fed-up, then don't do it for them. Do it for the little kid that you used to be, that kid who once had **BIG** dreams and imagination. The child that you were before the world had something to do with it. Before they stole your imagination and curiosity. That child who saw this great big world with wide-eyed wonder and awe of possibility. Now you're an adult in constant fear, frustration and dead-end cycles. You owe it to who you were, to be the hero for yourself now, that you needed then.

I am here to tell you that however you have been taught to live, if you are miserable and "stuck" and you feel that you belong there or deserve it, you have been taught wrong.

There very well may be a long season that you have been in because you didn't know better or didn't have tools to get out, but it is just that… a season. Your season of hardship doesn't define who you are, just like your moments of glory don't define you; how you live and treat yourself and others consistently day-to-day, *that* is who you are. How you receive and respond to your hardships and temporary successes, *that* is what defines you.

So, let's talk about it.

The hard parts too.

Because that is where we will find freedom and healing, not in running to other humans or substances or other addictions or distractions to escape or numb our pain or lack of connection, but in *facing* them head-on.

I want to face your demons with you and give you tools and hold your hand as you navigate through your darkness and find new light—for good.

I can't promise you that after reading this, you won't ever have times of deep sadness or discontentment, that isn't what this is about; I cannot take away your pain. However, I can promise to provide you with a different perception of your sadness and heaviness, so that you can turn your adversities and struggles into fire in your soul, rather than feeling like they're constantly going to drown you.

You may not agree with everything that is written, and that is fine. Some of it may be very new to you in a way that may have never been taught or said to you until now. You may wriggle around in your chair at the discomfort of awareness it brings you to read some of these deep, unknown truths...

But YOU are worth reading this with an open mind, then making the practical changes in your thoughts and actions to live a far more fulfilling life.

To live a bare minimum life, just to pay your bills and "get by" without having something bigger to contribute towards or something more satisfying to aim for; to only crave an acceptance into your own version of your Heaven *after* this lifetime, that is the lowest-level of gift to ask and strive for.

What if your gift of life **IS** your choice to be in Heaven or Hell while you're *here*, and your free will is your power and overall authority to decide which one you will live in?

Soak in this for a minute.

This isn't the kind of book you should rush through, please immerse yourself in what I am saying to you.

What if there *is no* Heaven or Hell after this?

What if this is it?

What if your afterlife is your reincarnation into your next life of Heaven or Hell *here* on Earth?

Who's to say that we aren't in Hell now? That no matter how "good" or "bad" of a person you are in this lifetime, you really screwed something up in the last one and now you're here to fix your mistake. Maybe it's up to *you* in this lifetime to complete a task that had been assigned to you several lifetimes ago and you haven't ever been able to figure it out, but each time you get sent back to start over, you get a little closer. What if there is no way out, other than overcoming the hard parts? When I was once in a really heavy place and having suicidal thoughts in the past, it has literally saved my life to stop and think that maybe if I take the "easy" way out, then I will just have to start right back over in the life that I was placed in now, but with new obstacles. My life has had a pattern of never rewarding my shortcuts long-term, so why would the Universe or my God bring me ease from taking the biggest shortcut of all in leaving my mission for them? Maybe I have been stuck in this same life for many lifetimes and it is *just now* that I am coming into awareness that I have to make deep-rooted, life-long lifestyle and soul changes in order to ever get out of this and come into more consistent light. Maybe the only way to ever permanently make it out of this Hell and get back home and stay there, is to master ourselves here, in order to bring our best there. Maybe your Universe wants you on a bigger mission than this miniscule human lifetime and your position of responsibility and leadership *there* is dependent on how you earned it *here.* Maybe, just maybe, if you can do what is necessary in this lifetime, even when it's really challenging, you will finally earn your way out of this.

Have you or your children ever played a video game?

In a lot of video games, there is a storyline with many tasks assigned to the player through countless lives and deaths, with the ultimate goal being to complete the game. You start as an "Infant Character," not knowing your way and dying for risks you'll eventually realize aren't safe. You'll have temporary highs, like Mario ingesting mushrooms that make him grow and feel more powerful, but eventually, something will always come along and knock him off his feet and shrink him back down to actual size - this doesn't mean defeat, this means you must be more cautious of obstacles as he moves forward in his weakened state. You'll gain awareness of the obstacles to come and you'll become more cautious and smarter about the decisions you make moving forward to the next obstacle. The challenges get harder, but you play more wisely. If you die along the way, you start over, but never ahead of where you died before. With this new chance at life moving forward, you have an edge on the enemy you'll face, because you use what you learned from your failed attempt at defeating it, and you approach them in a smarter, stronger way this time. Enough of these deaths and coming back to life, you'll die less and less and be prepared for obstacles based on your history, rather than needing signs for what's to come. Eventually, if you stay consistent and use the past lessons you learned, in order to do and be better, you'll beat the game. The same concept of life and death applies to the choices in your own progression that you make; take as long as you'd like to learn, but wouldn't you rather beat the game more quickly and with more efficiency? Every time you overcome an obstacle in this lifetime, you'll level up and unlock new powers that you never even knew you had; you'll also reveal new, bigger obstacles you'll have to conquer in order to move forward! These adversities are a gift in the process of you building your strength and power, as the ultimate defeat of the next enemy you face will require the tools you acquired from the last demon you slayed. In your true existence, at times it feels as if you dug yourself out of a hole, to crawl your way up a tall mountain, to discover a Goliath at the top. This game doesn't let you have long-term rest at the end of each level, you rest when you reach victory at the end of the game. Rest is necessary in the balance of your growth and development; however, you should never be looking forward to rest as a destination! What would be the purpose of continual rest?

I hear so many humans talk about reaching retirement, then when I ask them why they're looking forward to it so much, their response is generally that they won't have to "work" anymore. A lot of them don't even have plans for their life after that. What will you be doing that makes you feel *better* and more fulfilled than your career did? Would it be possible to live those more fulfilling ways before retirement? If who or where you receive your paycheck from isn't aligned with your values long-term, you should be leaving their employment behind long before your "retirement." To plan a retirement at the end of your planned career is a disrespect to your God, as if He/She doesn't have their own plan for you already. Who is to say your plans will be the same? Have your plans always carried a perfect track record for working out, or did it happen the way it was meant to, out of your control? What if God's plan for you doesn't include your plans? Live how you're craving so deeply to live *right now*, find joy and fulfillment and purpose *now*. If your soul has convicted you of a blessing that you know to be yours, don't place restrictions on the timeframe in which it will be delivered to you, based on your idea of when it should be. Don't minimize or second guess the power of your God.

You can have whatever belief system you'd like and believe in whichever afterlife you desire, but you really don't know *where* it will take place. What Heaven and Hell happen to be, have nothing to do with what you *assume* them to be.

Let's change our perception of feeling like these challenges are personal attacks sent to destroy us, to the understanding that they are actually here to help develop us and sharpen us into becoming the kind of being that can face ANYthing that expectedly or unexpectedly presents itself to us as challenge, with the knowledge that it is here to *better* you, not entrap you.

"My life keeps putting me through this over and over, it must just be trying to teach me something. Everything happens for a reason."

This is partly true. Your life does send you very clear lessons and assignments; it is up to you to acknowledge them, accept them and act on them right away - the *first* time. However, your Universe only wants to have to teach you **once**. *YOU choose* to keep yourself in a cycle of learning the same lessons over and over by not changing your thoughts and actions once you are convicted to make a change. Your life around and outside of you is not to blame for your cycles, *you are.*

"Life is *hard.*"

"Healing is *hard.*"

"Growth is *hard.*"

"I have *no* reason to live."

I know, I know...

"Right when you open your eyes to your day, there are countless-endless things presented to your being to keep you in your complacency, sadness and hopelessness." Right?

And you are somewhat right.

You are without a doubt, faced with all this each day if you choose to see it that way.

But what if we changed our view even a little and just switched small words we are used to, to more purposeful, less generalized ones?

Like changing the word *hard* to *challenging.*

Hard seems so daunting and miserable to approach, when really the *challenges* that are presented to us, are there to open our eyes to something and to teach us, in hopes that we will listen to our Universe and make changes accordingly - they aren't here to victimize us.

The first step in becoming the best version of yourself is accepting responsibility for who you are today. Rather than being a victim of your circumstances, forgive yourself for not knowing or doing better before, and move forward with enough confidence and love for yourself. You KNOW you deserve better from you, regardless of how you've treated yourself in the past.

These changes will be uncomfortable and challenging at times, but they will save you lifetimes of dead-end cycles and give you access to the power you never even realized you had inside of you all this time.

Trauma looks different to each individual soul; don't minimize your hardship because of the challenges of others around you not looking the same as yours. If experiences of your past hurt you, or changed you, or affected who you are today, they matter. They deserve to be addressed, handled and healed from. The hardships that have happened in your upbringing to this point do not deserve to take any more of your life and love than they have already taken.

You deserve freedom from yourself.

You're worth looking into this mirror.

Please take your time reading this book. Give yourself some grace, patience, and lots of repented forgiveness as you peel back layers of yourself you may be meeting for the first time.

As you read this book, talk within yourself, as if you *are* the Mother you've always needed, conversing with the childhood version of you, as the adult you are in this moment.

CHAPTER 1: YOUR TRUTH VS. THEIRS

Regardless of who or what was around you the moment you popped out of your mama, you showed up into this world *all alone*, at your very particular, special time of arrival - planned or not.

And you will *leave* the same way.

(One of those 'wriggle in your chair' truths, when you stop and soak in it.)

What happens between those two dates of arrival, that is entirely up to you.

Despite our differences of upbringing, we all share more in common than you think…

None of us got to choose to be here, we didn't choose our parents or most of our teachers, how or where we were raised, our beliefs, our means of education, our nutrition, etc. All these decisions were made for us and we were required to live these ways in order to appease others that were in control of us. A lot of times, if we rebelled against their standard, even if we felt convicted to do so, we would be punished or disciplined into behaving "correctly" according to their lifestyle. There was a "perfect picture" for your family to present to everybody else, the ones that didn't get to see all the dysfunction behind the scenes, right?

I treat children (even the grown ass, snotty ones) with a lot more grace, patience and kindness now, because I've realized that children aren't "naughty," they are curious, and they make mistakes and they are learning. And, more often than not, a lot of them are being misguided and mislead by parents that never took the time to heal their soul on the *inside*, before they became responsible for part of their soul being *outside* of them. Guys, this results in adult assholes that are just grown children that never healed from their (or their parents') past traumas and false teachings.

Whenever I see an adult throw an actual real life fit, I legitimately picture them as a child whose mom didn't give them their way and they don't know how to control their emotions and never cared to learn. I've had grown men come up to my counter at a pizza restaurant I worked at who were bright red in the face, with veins comin' out of their neck, shouting about not having the flavor of pizza they prefer on our buffet. My managers, co-workers and friends would always come grab me to diffuse a situation because I always found such humor and opportunity in a grown being throwing a fit over something that bares such little significance in their Big Picture. I would always approach the situation with a smile and open heart, because I knew the real issue really had nothing to do with the pizza at all. They're hurting about something and a pizza restaurant employee is an easy target to use as a disconnected punching bag. I would let them vent for a moment without taking any of it personally, then would say with a chuckle, something along the lines of, "Listen, I have no idea what is going on in your life outside of this building, but I'm so sorry for your pain. The least I can do for you is make you the pizza you're looking for, but you owe my co-worker an apology for treating them that shitty when they're just here trying to make a living for their family like you and I are." I am not even exaggerating when I say that most of the time, they would be apologetic and taken back, even sometimes brought to tears. I treat them in the same way I would've treated my eight-year-old daughter, it's all the same.

You see, regardless of how you were raised, this incredible shift eventually happens in your life one day when you'll have the choice to live whichever lifestyle you choose. You get to separate yourself from your upbringing as much as you desire and decide for yourself what this life will be. You get the free will to make the decision to live for your own happiness and joy and fulfillment, just like they do. You get to sit down with yourself and your Universe and decide what you believe in, which relationships you will invest in, and what your day-to-day joys will consist of.

I was taught this brilliant Task of Clarity:

There is a tool to write in at the end of this book, or you can get a blank sheet of paper and separate it into two sections: One section titled "What I have Been Taught," and the other titled, "What I Believe." Underneath "What I Have Been Taught," write down anything and everything that you have ever been taught or told or shown an example of in your life as a way of living, whether you agree with it or not. (Who have you been told that you are? What have you been taught you can achieve, not achieve? What will your future consist of? What insecurities do you have?)

Now, on the other side, "What I Believe," write down what you actually believe in! Not based on anybody else's words, judgements or expectations.

Who you believe you are at your best, *that* is who you are.

If you're in a season of not being your best self, that is *not* who you are. Your *beliefs* are who you are. Who you will be at your best, *that* is who you are.

So, it is imperative that you figure out for yourself what it is that you believe in. Then you stand up for those beliefs with conviction and authority, every single chance that you get. Defend your beliefs through your actions and your testimonies of overcoming; protect your beliefs through your self-respect and self-love and express them with confidence. Your Universe will respond to and deliver to you more of what you are confident and secure in. Going back to changing our definitions in order to make progress: I learned recently that if you live a life of pleasing others, you are not a "people-pleaser," you are a "value-sacrificer."

We must stop focusing so much on treating the dysfunctional symptoms of the world like substance and alcohol addiction, anti-socialism, suicide rates on the constant rise, depression, or lack of parenting, etc., and start focusing more on fixing the roots that *create* those symptoms! Don't get me wrong, these are all truly devastating and awful issues, but the entire reason we have all these *symptoms* is because of a much deeper epidemic of lost, disconnected humans that don't know what to stand for anymore.

"We have a human collective following rules that they don't believe in, to appease humans that don't even contribute to their happiness in any consistent way anyways, resulting in lives they are unhappy and unsatisfied with."

Once the deep-rooted feelings of hopelessness set in, we can't figure out why, and/or we don't know how to fix it, so we seek anything we can that will temporarily make us numb or distract us from our pain. Then we feel guilty for digging ourselves deeper into our self-harming hole while we were hurting, so we pull it together for a while, realizing that a temporary high wasn't the answer. Once we try our hardest to not relapse into defeat and *that* doesn't work, we end up in a cycle of running right back to the temporary fix that made us feel better for even just a moment.

We have a human collective addicted to temporary highs, no matter the cost of our long-term health and stability. The more our over-all stability suffers through our lack of purpose and distractions, the more we crave the temporary, destructive highs. Substance and alcohol are just some of the most apparent forms of a high that we are suffering from a lack of control of. This isn't just some substance issue, we have also become more consumed with comparison and outside approval than ever before! Social media attention has become more valued to us than our own family's attention and security. Having a nicer truck than John, or a bigger house than Jane is worth more than our family's long-term financial safety and stability. A certain number of "likes" has become more assuring to our self-worth than a compliment from our spouse or loved one.

All temporary highs.

No amount of "likes" online will ever express to you your *actual* value or worth. Social media attention is like the Monopoly® money of Love Languages.

Pay attention to actual, relevant ways that the Universe hits the "like" button on your life. If you pay close enough attention, your life will actually "like" your efforts by offering you a hand up, or genuine gifts.

Green lights the entire way to work when you're running behind.

A compliment from a stranger.

A random credit to your finances.

Assistance without asking for it, in a time of need.

A good night's rest for the first time in a very long time.

Etc.

These are *all* Universe "likes".

The list can be endless literally daily, if you choose to acknowledge it. They are everywhere every day, and you'll see them right away if you exert as much time, attention and focus into finding them, as you do your social media search for approval and attention. The more life "likes" you recognize and feel and show *gratitude* towards, the more "likes" are sent! Just as if you never showed yourself on social media, you would have nothing for anybody to have the opportunity to "like," if you never show up in your life, your life has no way of sending you "likes."

The Universe is literally begging to help you, but it can't guide your steps if you aren't willing to walk into the life you've been promised.

"Nobody in this world is better than you. And nobody is worse."

We are all equal in this, no matter what our upbringing, no matter the difference of our gifts. Nobody has what you dream of because they "deserve" better than you. Some people have a lot of really cool shit and don't deserve any of it - that doesn't make them any better than you. You may have a lot of cool shit yourself, that doesn't make you any better than the person standing next to you that happens to be in a different season of their story. Worldly possessions are even more temporary than our existence here, they can vanish in an instant, then what do you have left when you don't have any more things? Are you still a *somebody* without your worldly accumulations?

If you have a pure heart with consistently loving intentions and you're constantly seeking ways to get better, that is worth infinite amounts more than any worldly, material possession will ever be! You already have a priceless, unshakeable treasure that cannot be taken away by anybody's authority other than your own; what comes into your worldly possession meanwhile, that is just a cherry on top of who and what you already *are*! As we had talked about before with rest, worldly possessions are only tools to help you in reaching your purpose, they should not *be* your ultimate purpose. You must reach a point of enough self-awareness and self-respect, that you would still feel 100% worthy and validated in being here and find pure value in your existence, even if you had nothing. Because you truly are more than *enough* all on your own.

If what you are doing day-to-day isn't in alignment with what you believe in, it is inevitably pulling you away from who you truly are. You will never, ever find yourself that way. You will find *yourself* in your renewed lifestyle of gratitude and Godly (Loving) connection and every thought and action you have being a testament to what you believe in.

Once you have established your renewed belief system, it is imperative for your process to *forgive* your **entire** past and *let it go*. You can carry the lessons with you for the rest of your life, but you must move forward from yesterday. You must forgive yourself first, for not knowing better, for not listening to your convictions or trusting them, for hurting yourself and for others mistakenly being hurt in the crossfires of your healing (or lack thereof), for not treating yourself with the love and respect you deserve, etc. In order to forgive yourself, you must take responsibility for where you are at this very moment of reading these words. There are a lot of circumstances that have been out of control of in your life, but the result of those circumstances has been completely up to you; you have zero control over the actions of others, but you are in full control of your response. Once you acknowledge that *you* are the one responsible for your every action and decision, you will realize that every single person around you has the exact same responsibility over *their* actions, too. Most of the times that you have really caused pain in others (intentionally, or not), have happened at times that you were in a lot of pain yourself. As humans, we inflict onto others the energies we *feel* internally, regardless of what we put on for show on the outside, or whether we mean to or not. When you feel your best and you are happy and at peace, you don't have any desire to inflict anything other than those traits onto those around you. Meaning, if somebody else treats you awfully, it is more than likely because they feel really awfully about something in their world, even if they haven't acknowledged it for themselves yet. If somebody treats you with unworldly kindness, that also has nothing to do with who you are, that is simply because that is how they feel, and they are exuding that energy onto you. If you really take time to think about it, this releases you from any past guilt you may have about the outcome of the pain you have inflicted on another soul; the pain you inflicted was not their choice by any means and you may have made a mistake in hurting them and that is totally on you, but how they chose to live after that is entirely up to them. They have the choice to use the pain you caused through your lack of understanding, as a tool for their growth, as well, if they choose to seek joy over self-victimization. You can acknowledge that you did wrong and apologize to them genuinely for hurting them, without attachment to responsibility for who they are today, or expectations of who they will be for you tomorrow. You can't change what you have done to harm yourself or those around you, but you can start doing better *now*. You can forgive yourself and you can forgive them by doing better and sharing with those around you how they can find light, too. Forgiveness is an inside job, that is all for you. You don't forgive others as a justification for what they did, you forgive others because you deserve freedom from the pain that they caused you. They must live with what they have done and handle it the way they choose, just as you have the responsibility to determine how you will move forward. Quit overthinking your past. You can't change or fix it; you can only learn and repent and grow from your mistakes and overcome them once and for all as you *accept them and move forward without attachment.*

"A mistake made more than once is a decision."

"The only way to heal a wound is to stop touching it," healing will not come from dissecting your faults. Healing begins with accepting your past, learning from it, then having an unquenchable desire to be better and to do better. Healing comes from perpetuating focus on building fueling relationships and connections with ourselves and the world around us today, so that inevitably, we crave those more than our temporary highs, tomorrow."

"And if I asked you of all of the things you loved most in this life, where would you be on that list?"

It's about time that you start treating yourself with the same kind of love with which you treated the person/thing you fell most in love with in your past. You are worth every bit of the love you have looked for so desperately outside of yourself.

CHAPTER 2: FINDING YOUR PURPOSE

It's all gotten so complicated. There has been so much societal pressure and judgement and rules and standards for our ideas of "success" and what our "purpose" in being here should be.

"Your purpose has nothing to do with what anybody else wants for you; your purpose is found in the same place as your passion and your love. If you have lost either of those, you have more than likely lost the other, because they are connected. If you have lost what you loved most and have not found something else to be productively passionate about, then you are probably feeling less than purposeful."

Your purpose is not found in your moments of success; you carry the same purpose, no matter which season you're in. Who are you between your successes, if your successes are what make you a *somebody?*

"The planet does not need more successful people. The planet desperately needs more peacemakers, healers, restorers, storytellers and lovers of all kinds." - Dalai Lama

If you're struggling with finding your purpose, maybe your purpose isn't *you.* Maybe your constant focus on yourself is distracting you from a bigger purpose of being able to be there for others. Maybe the battles you have faced on your path were there to strengthen you to fight for others on theirs.

Your purpose can be found over time by incorporating new things into each day that *feel* good. Maybe you don't know what your purpose outside of today is, but **today** has purpose for *you*. Regardless of how you feel, the *fact* is that life isn't meant to feel heavy or miserable. Why not start with one of the simplest, yet hardest to master purposes of all - just to *feel* good consistently, long-term? It is one of the saddest facts of life to me, how many humans go through their entire life without even knowing what it's like to just *feel* good. It is such an injustice to the miracle of your existence to go through life without knowing what you're capable of, to feel obligated to live, rather than feeling the warmth of life with the gratitude overtaking the depths of your lungs with each breath you take.

Every single thing you do in your life will either contribute to your purpose or pull you away from it, there is no in between; what you watch, what you read, what you eat and drink, who and what you surround yourself with, **all** of it. Your purpose is not found in temporary highs, it is found in what brings you long-term peace and joy. How is what you're doing today contributing positively to who you will be tomorrow?

If you're deeply lost and sad and don't want to be in this existence anymore, if you have ever thought about ending your life, commit a *living* suicide. Die to yourself and who you used to be and start over... while you're *alive*... because remember, dying for real will potentially make you have to start completely over and that would be absolutely defeating. Suicide, to me, is not a permanent escape, it's a "false reset" button and you start over in the same life as an infant again. But, in a living suicide, you get to die to your past and *still* have **all** that wisdom you have acquired over this lifetime. You get to start back at a checkpoint in your Life Video Game; much more of an advantage and opportunity to make a more permanent change that way. Who would you be, if you considered yourself to be invisible to others and untouchable in any way emotionally, as if you were an Angel roaming the Earth in bliss? Picture yourself as an Angel; nothing could touch you in a negative way anymore, because you don't live for your feelings anymore, Angels are only love. You don't get to think negative thoughts anymore, Angels are only love. At this point, you only get to contribute and allow contribution of love to your existence, the rest of it, you have chosen to be repellant of. If you don't have something positive to add to others, you start working on positive things to add to your own days and let those manifest.

After your living suicide, you will dissect everything that comes into your path day-by-day. Does it serve you joy? Does it make you cheek-sore smile or laugh? Will you feel good about this decision tomorrow? Does it align with who you want to be and will be? Every single decision you make will pull you out of the hole or put you deeper into it.

It's imperative to your long-term health and wellness to not mask your sadness with substance, addiction, distraction or fear, but to face it and soak in it and make sense of it as much as you can as you progress. Your sadness is not meant to be a destination, neither is your singleness or your hardships. But they all serve a deep *purpose*. Without the dark, heavy stuff, we would have a much harder time appreciating and being grateful for the light.

"The deeper you take care of the roots, the stronger the winds and storms it can endure!"

Challenges don't ever stop in life. Right when you overcome one obstacle, guess what, there will be an even bigger one waiting for you after your victory. That's what happens when you reach a new level. You don't get to choose all the battles you face, but you do get to decide how you will spend your time preparing for them. You were dropped off into a battlefield down here, my friends. You must pick a side. You **cannot** become complacent on this battlefield; your life will stampede over you! Use these challenges to sharpen your weapons, so you more than just *make it out*, but you slay every single damn thing that tries to get in your way, with a legion following your example because of what they have seen you overcome and stand up for.

Every single thing that you do in this life will either provide strength and support and guidance for battle, or it will help in your demise. You must armor yourself in confidence and authority in your beliefs and your mission each day before you ever even leave your home. You must sharpen your weapons, put on your armor and know how to fight for yourself.

"Iron Sharpens Iron So One Man Sharpens Another." Proverbs 27:17

Surround yourself with other warriors of similar beliefs. If you aren't sharpening your blades, you are inevitably dulling them.

Offer other soldiers that are down, a hand-up, but not at the expense of your own safety or well-being.

Rest. When the time is right. Not for too long, but when your mind and body have told you it is time, knowing that the *purpose* isn't to get comfortable and stay there, you're only there to recover.

Acknowledge that this battle will not end, so long as you are here. You are here to represent a side in a battle of good vs. evil, and I can tell you that you were *not* born to be evil, this hell on Earth is turning people against who they were born to be. You were born with compassion and grace and strength and endless capability and love; evil is only acquired through lack of love and light and understanding. The focus isn't for us to remove the dark, but instead, fight back with light. Love will always win.

FIGHT!

If you have felt at times, that you are all alone in this... I am here to tell you that you *are*.

Pretty devastating, right??

Wrong.

How *freeing*.

You don't owe anybody a single, damn thing.

You don't *belong* to anybody or anything other than your Creator.

You are enough, all on your own. Even if you can't stand to be alone with yourself right now.

BY KALEY CAMARE

You are powerful and capable and have made it to this point and these pages all alone, no matter who has or hasn't chosen to stick by your side along the way. As a matter of fact, thank God for the people that were honest enough to walk away, rather than sticking around to continue dulling your blade with their ingenuine or selfish use of your relationship. You deserve to be loved deeply, passionately, faithfully - by yourself first... And then, to not accept an ounce less than that from anybody outside of you. You are better off loving yourself, over having somebody around that makes you feel like you are hard to love.

In order to fulfill our bigger-picture purpose, whatever it may be, even if it *is* just to feel good, we must focus on the alignment of that with our daily purposes. *Everything* should be done with intention and on *purpose.* If it doesn't serve your bigger picture or beliefs for yourself, it doesn't deserve even a minimal amount of your attention, positive or negative. What time did you wake up this morning? What purpose did that serve to awake then? If you woke up early, maybe it was because you have a job to be at because you have a livelihood to provide for, or because you had to get your kiddo to an extracurricular activity, maybe it was so that you could have some *you* time to soak up the Universe before the rest of your day comes at you. *Maybe* it was very purposeful for you to wake up that early. Or maybe you slept in today. What was the purpose in that? Perhaps you have been struggling with sleep lately and this was the *one* morning of the week you were able to make up for lost rest and there was *purpose* in that. But if you only sleep in longer than necessary out of a lifestyle habit or laziness and it's more sleep than your human needs and is stealing time from your days that you could be maximizing sharpening your blade, then it doesn't serve a *purpose* and it then must to be confronted, battled and overcome! You have ultimate control and authority in your life; small accumulated acts of finding daily purpose is what will help you to rediscover your confidence and power.

What is your nutrition like? What purpose does it serve? Is it fueling your human body's necessities for survival, or are you feeding your misleading and ever-changing feelings?

Who are you spending your time in the presence of? Are they in alignment with your bigger-picture purpose, or are they just fun and distracting *today*? Do they support you and sharpen you, or is misery just a really big fan of your company because it knows you've been too weak to leave? Are they good to you *now,* or just potentially?

Everything serves a purpose, either to help you in your battle, or to distract you. Choose your *purposes* wisely.

As a child, you would ask, "Why? Why? Why?" Over and over about anything and everything because you were genuinely so curious about the *purpose* behind things. Your "Why's" were eventually silenced because whomever was asked either didn't want to answer or didn't have an answer themselves. You must reclaim your "Why." Every single thing you are doing. Why?? Is it benefiting you long-term in some way, are you helping somebody without causing yourself long-term suffering, is what you're doing aligned with your beliefs? If not, then put it to an end immediately. It's more than okay to ask, "Why?" As a matter of fact, it is imperative that you *do.*

Every single thing you encounter in your day:

"Why am I doing this?"

"Why am I consuming this?"

"Why am I in this particular person's presence?"

You must be in constant reflection of your purpose and whether your actions are aligned. If your actions don't serve your purpose, you must change your actions, in order to prevent the sacrificing of becoming who you are destined to be.

CHAPTER 3: RELATIONSHIPS

No single way that you are feeling is a coincidence. Whether it be a small headache or a deep sadness, or the opposition of having great feelings, or a "gut feeling" about something, it all has roots. And like I have said previously, at the very least, you weren't meant to feel anything less than your best. There are actual, practical lifestyle habits that contribute to how you feel, both positively and negatively. *Everything* effects how you feel. And as human beings, we have a relationship with literally everything we come into the presence of: our other human loves, our career, our Creator, what we consume, our vehicles, our bodies, strangers we encounter, nature and animals, etc.

What are your relationships like?

Are you aware of them?

Do they serve your beliefs, or pull you away from them?

Have you neglected, or served them? Have you seen the correlation in their relationship back with you?

The more intentional focus you put on something, the more love and light and effort you pour into growing your relationship with that specific thing, the more it will inevitably grow. And if it doesn't, you must take all that love, light and effort to a place where it will grow.

If you feel lonely, this isn't a coincidence or a feeling that you should just "shake off" either, however it's possible that it isn't for the reasons that you think; loneliness only comes from a place of not finding 100% comfort in your own company. And if *you* aren't comfortable being around you, why would anybody else be? I'm not talking about isolation, that only sinks you further into sadness, I'm talking about *alone time.* Just as life wasn't meant to feel constantly heavy, it also wasn't meant to be lived alone, however, *alone time* is necessary to be able to serve the relationships outside of us the best we can. You were meant for relationships, like I said before, your daily life is made up of them with everything you encounter, whether you like it or not. Your lack of participation doesn't prevent the battle from prevailing; if you don't choose your relationships, they will inevitably choose you.

How is your relationship with yourself? How do you speak to yourself, take care of yourself, present yourself to the world? Your relationship with yourself will help to create your identity; what is it that you will identify as? I picture in my living suicide, having an actual service for myself and the birds-eye view of how everybody would respond to my death, as if it were the real thing. I play it out in my head. I have those close to me that would be very devastated; some would be expressive, and some would go into silence, but it would *affect* them, because I have touched their life in some way. Some would show up to my service because they feel obligated, or out of support for my other loves there. Some would show up and talk to the others, as if we were best friends, even though we haven't even spoken since I was young. Some would make it about them, and some wouldn't come at all. But, when I do leave this state of being, the funeral service that they have won't be for me, I will already be gone and at peace; it will be for *them.* For them to support each other in their personal loss, to grieve, to gain closure, etc. You see, even your very own death is not about *you* to the outside world, so why would you expect the world outside of you to take care of you while you're here? They're all busy trying to make sure *they* are fulfilling *their* mission here, not yours. A lot of people want to end their life, without even having an ideal life they'd like to be experiencing in mind. So, what if instead of committing a "living death" to yourself like we talked about, you actually did commit a death suicide, and because the Universe didn't plan that for you, it starts you back over where you started this last time and *this* existence is actually your hell that *you* have to find your way out of? So, if you had to start over and your outcome was 100% up to you, what would you have done differently? What people/places would you dig into *more* and which places and people and things would you pay no mind to at all? Why do you have to die for real, in order to experience that kind of control over your destiny and make necessary changes to acquire joy? You can literally do that right now in a single moment… while you're still here, alive and feeling. Wanting to die only comes from a place of not knowing how to *live* for yourself, rather than the world outside of you.

What are your relationships like with the humans around you? Your close loves, your children, your spouse, co-workers, etc.?

What expectations do you have of each of the people you're in relationships with? If they had the exact same expectations of you, would you be fulfilling them?

Are you in relationships with them solely based on what they can do to serve you, or do you also have a desire to add light to their life intentionally, too? A life of gaining from everybody else with little payment of your love to others, may allow for you to gain temporary relationships and worldly possessions, but will inevitably leave you very lonely and unfulfilled long-term.

Maybe you have experienced the alternative of having a lot of relationships that you felt you gave everything to, but never received a fair amount of love or care in return. The great news is, love will always find its way home, it just isn't up to us which form it is delivered in. No amount of love is ever wasted, even if it isn't utilized by who is directly being loved. The more love you put out into the world, the more love will find you in ways you never expected. The same goes for anything else you exude to the outside world, positive or negative - it will all find its way back to you on the Universe's timeline. The key isn't to stop giving your love away because it wasn't received correctly, the key is to learn when to invest your love elsewhere, upon awareness of it not growing where you've placed it. Awareness and action are everything. Sticking around to help somebody isn't always loving them, as much as it is enabling them. Trying to keep somebody away from their pain and being resentful about how they are unable to love you in return is such a disservice to their growth and self-love; it only allows them to keep perpetuating their wrong way of living and loving.

As a living being that needs several types of fuel for life, let's take a moment to envision you as a plant within your own planter-pot. In order to not only sustain life, but to grow and to thrive, too, you require the proper care. Not only do you need the proper nutrients, but you need the proper environment and balance of those nutrients, as well. With the right care, with the correct forms of fuel and a good consistent dose of light and warmth, your roots will expand and grow, resulting in a thriving, blossoming plant. Your plant requires this process of care eternally, as long as it lives, or it will inevitably die. In most cases, unless something unexpectedly traumatic and sudden happens, your plant wouldn't die immediately, it would be a process of neglect and mistreatment that led it to its wilted demise. Now, I want you to understand something... When you enter a relationship with somebody or something outside of yourself, you are inviting that plant to reside inside of your planter with you. Once this other plant is planted next to you, in your nutrient-dense soil and under your same warm light, its roots will begin to grow and merge with yours. This is where your awareness becomes vital. Once your roots merge, you will inevitably begin to share life and take life from each other while pulling from each other's energies. It is imperative that you are very careful of who/what you invite into your safe space (planter), as it will either bring you to more life, or it will drain you of your life altogether. This process doesn't happen in a catastrophic moment, this is the process of an extended time of ignoring seemingly insignificant signs of death. As humans, we need to become more aware of when life is being stolen from our roots, long before our plants are wilted away. With the right plants planted next to you, your roots will multiply and grow and flourish, creating life so rapidly and vigorously, that your growth becomes unstoppable! In opposition, once you're in awareness that there is a plant next to you draining the life from your roots, you should feed it an extra dose love and care and see if it will come back into consistent life, but if it doesn't, you must detach their roots from yours and let them take from life somewhere that doesn't continue to take from yours. You can still love the way that plant looks, feels and lives from a distance, all while not allowing it to steal any more life from you.

More of a finance person?

If you had invested a large amount of money into something and rather than making your money grow, it cost you each month, and your funds decreased… would you keep putting money into it? Or would you pull your funds and place them into a different investment that you could grow your finances from? It's the same concept with your love. If you bankrupt yourself, it isn't *their* fault, it's yours. You bankrupting your love didn't happen overnight, it happened a little bit at a time, each time you took a failed relationship personally, every time you made a mistake and didn't forgive yourself and repent and do better, you not accepting when it was time to walk away and remaining in these cycles over and over, etc. These heartaches that have depleted your love account were not *their* fault. The initial infliction of pain that they caused may have been out of your control and may have really hurt you and cost you, but how you have responded and adapted to the pain, *those* are love funds that *you* are responsible for replenishing or draining. You are not required to show any human being walking this Earth (other than your children) more love than you show yourself-but you *are* required to love yourself, in order to live peacefully and joyously and with long-term fulfillment. The more you can invest into your self-love account, the more funds you will have to give away. If you're feeling a little drained and defeated, odds are your love account just needs replenished. You may be a couple dollars short, or you may be in debt up to your ears in loss of love, but the only way to recover from that is to start making deposits every chance that you can! Stop withdrawing funds that you don't have; your love debt could be the death of you. Once you have attained wealth in love, don't just keep it all to yourself, share it with those around you that invest in you, too. Watch the love manifest right in front of you, once you start investing it in the right places.

It is imperative that you know that a season that you are growing through, does *not* define who you are. Do not let sadness or complacency take away your entire life. Your feelings are not true.

Depression is a very real feeling, it isn't just some cooked up thought that will eventually leave you alone, but that doesn't make it a fact. It isn't something that masks of pills, substances, other addictions, or distractions will ever treat. If you were up against your opponent in battle and they had prepared for your defeat knowing all you had as a weapon against them was a bottle of pills or booze that *they* gave to you, they would laugh in your face and then hunt you the hell down because you're much easier to attack when you're phased. Overcoming deep sadness, just like any other opponent you face, takes intense, deliberate *war*! It takes the most strength and grit you have ever freaking felt. There are times it will take every bit of what you have practiced your entire life to muster the strength to defeat it. You will crawl across the floor with nowhere to go and STILL get back up, because you learned to trust that voice inside of you saying, **"GET UP!"** There isn't a human or substance that can permanently rid you of the feeling.

The only thing that will get you out of any awful way that you are stuck feeling, is to separate your *feelings* from the *facts.*

Feelings are real, but they are not *true*; feelings are ever-changing. Facts are always the same and never change. Feelings are based on individual perception, whereas facts are the same, no matter what the perception. When you come into any feeling, good or bad, determine if it contributes positively to your battle long-term by separating the facts from how you are feeling, then *always* live by the facts. Accept and *soak* in your feelings when they come, but then determine *why* you feel this way. Maybe it's justified, but maybe it *isn't.*

"I am just so depressed today."

Okay. When you're hungry, you eat. You don't just sit there playing victim about it until you die of starvation. When you're cold, you find something to keep you warm, you don't just sit there and cry about it until you freeze to death. Sadness is an *actual* feeling, so how do you *fix* it, rather than just being a victim of it? First, acknowledge that this is a changeable *feeling*, it isn't *who you are.* Have the understanding that it's okay to be sad, but you can still get shit done at the same time. Sadness isn't a death sentence, it's just a season that you will overcome. Get up. Take a shower, wash off all that sad baggage. Dress yourself up a little more than your "sad" clothes, but not in anything too tight. Get outside, even if it's for a 10-minute walk around the block. Organize just *one* area of your life - your nightstand, your phone contacts, your black hole of a closet or purse, just *something.* Treat yourself with grace and patience in your time of healing, don't put pressure on needing to *feel* better. Put one foot in front of the other, healing will come in the fight, not in the fold.

Your identity is who you are at your best.

A great friend of mine was once heavily addicted to meth and a lifestyle of constant highs by way of running from the law and getting away with as many of those temporary highs as possible. Life was boring without it, the 9-5 was his idea of Hell. He didn't like authority and didn't want to have to answer to anybody, and that lifestyle happened to provide that for him. He didn't have the tools to know better at that point. He *felt* addicted to the rush, he didn't ever want to land in prison or hurt anybody or cause trouble, he just craved that *feeling* so badly. Unfortunately, this lifestyle finally caught up with him. After he was done with his prison time, he got out and remained sober and was determined to find a new lifestyle that served the *purpose* of giving him those same rushes, without the negative backlash. The facts of his lifestyle outweighed his feeling to continue using drugs and living that lifestyle, so he found a lifestyle that would provide that same feeling but be more sustainable and fulfilling in a balanced way. He got a job working on the oil rigs two weeks on, then two weeks off. He says the two weeks on, he is focused and planning his two weeks off and it feels a bit how prison did, and he uses it to dig into his mind, then two weeks a month he has complete freedom to do whatever he wants. His highs of choice now: running in the Ironman Challenges, deep-sea fishing, travelling, climbing 14ers. Getting rushes from his exploration and adventures; it works for him.

It's okay to not want to be like everybody else or live the way you were raised or like anybody around you but let the way you choose to live be a testament to your beliefs. There is no compromise here.

What do you seek from your relationships with others?

Are you expectant of something from other humans that you should be giving to yourself first?

Get out a sheet of paper. Write down everything that you desire out of a relationship with whom you want to share your life. What does your dream relationship look like? Whether you are in a relationship, or not, write what non-negotiable expectations you have of who you desire to be with. NOT expectations based on who you're with or who has damaged you in the past, yet based on what you truly desire for your day-to-day now and to your big picture future.

Once you have written your list, go over every expectation you have written and determine if you are fulfilling those for *yourself.*

Are *you* treating yourself to that level of standards? If not, then you have no right to hold anybody in your life to those standards of loving you until you can teach them the level in which to love you by showing them yourself! If you aren't loving yourself correctly, how can you love anybody else with your purest form of love, if you haven't discovered it or explored it for yourself yet?

Once you can confidently check off each expectation you are fulfilling on your list for yourself, you can then determine if who you are pursuing aligns with your highest form of love for yourself and gratitude for the life God has given you. You must take your *feelings* out of it and look at your **facts.**

Love is action.

If who you're pursuing in hopes for a life with them doesn't consistently **add** to the incredible amount of love you should already have for yourself, then you must let them go.

You are worth and deserve the love you are so desperate to seek.

May you desperately seek that love within yourself and let your God and Universe only deliver the kinds of love that add light and strength to your path.

Are you somebody whose relationships are there more consistent "failures" than loves that you can keep in your path?

If you are stuck in a cycle of relationships always ending, to a point in which it is almost expected before it ever even presents itself to you, you have some roots to tend to. Your failed relationships and lack of growth through them didn't start in your twenties, it started when you were a child. What were your relationships with your parents like? What affected you and changed you when you were a little, more impressionable version of yourself? How did your parents love you that you wish to extend to others? How did your parents *not* see you, what did they *do* or *not do* that defined love for you? Regardless of who you were raised by, or how you were raised, we all have our own version of our trauma that is incomparable to the trauma experienced by any other person. We are *all* victims of *something*, if we choose to look at it that way. We all have our own demons that come against us that we must fight, you can't allow your ego to minimize or put a Band-Aid® on the experiences that affected you growing up, whether anybody else understands them, or not. Your pain and heartache and loss are valid, and though it wasn't deserved, it holds an extremely valuable purpose for who you are becoming. You must accept what has happened, but not by casting it out of your mind and distracting yourself from it; you must forgive those that harmed you, so that you can forgive yourself for your inherited habit of self-sabotage. I now have this belief that we're all doing our best, even if all of our bests don't always look the same. And with hard work and a whole lot of love, our best will continually get even better, so that we can *do* and *be* better for ourselves and the existence around us.

My parents did the best they could, they loved all eight of us kids from the very deepest parts of their hearts, yet I still grew up with trauma. If you could rewind our past and play each of our childhoods, as if it were a movie trailer, they would all look very different, even growing up in the same household. We all grew up and we each handled our trauma differently. Some of us were able to forgive and break chains to detach from our trauma, some of us have fallen down a rabbit hole of empty highs and unsustainable life choices. And that is okay, I still love each of them even more so than when we were kids together, because I understand why they are who they are, even if it doesn't justify it. You see, you don't get to choose all the hardships that come into your path, just like you don't have control of your blessings, however, you do get to choose how you utilize your experiences, both good and bad. You can make the choice to use your pain as a tool. You can be inflicted with harm, yet still be detached from feeling victimized through gratitude of the awareness it has brought you, so that you can now create proper boundaries. You can still love people whose hearts beat differently than yours, just maybe not the way you had expected or pictured to love them in your mind. Not everybody loves the same way you do, and you can't hold that against them; you can only make a choice to accept them or let them find a love that will.

One of, if not the biggest grievance of my life, was the loss of my longest-term, most attached relationship I had been in. The one that I had poured the most of my raw self into, the one that I was 100% certain would lead to marriage and raising our children together, the one that I was so sure would last, that I took every moment of it for granted. We had both gone through a lot of struggle and growth together, within our own individual lives, and as a team and family. We both put each other through our own versions of heaven and hell over years of time. And, one day she had enough of the inconsistencies, and she drew her boundary and she left. I knew she would be back, like usual. She seemed pretty serious, so I knew that maybe this time would be longer than the last, but inevitably, she would be back to us. Man, my ego then. After all, she was mine. Leaving wasn't even an option, right? The first gut-wrenching days went by, then weeks, then months. She didn't come back. I saw her and for the first time since the breakup, I told her how awful I was without her, that I needed her in my life and I didn't know how to handle it and that I was sure it would be the death of me! Her response was very calm and detached, "I don't even know what to do for you anymore." And, that was it; I was shocked. She wasn't there anymore, and that was the first time I felt her actually gone right in front of me. Not on Facebook with another person, not the day she left, but the moment she was no longer my safe place, not even as a friend.

In the following months, she got serious with another woman and later became happily engaged, and is living a joyous, fulfilled life. It took me years of wondering what was wrong with me, why I wasn't worthy, what I was doing wrong and analyzing the details and trying to "figure" it all out, to finally realize through her newfound happiness, our hearts simply didn't beat the same. Sure, we put each other through A LOT of incredible high highs and a lot of incredibly low lows, but I never could sustain her, or her me. Though we wronged each other in our own traumatic ways, neither of us was the bad guy. Neither of us are bad people or wish anything less than love for each other, our hearts simply just crave different lifestyles and depths of love. And that is okay. I am so happy for who she decided to become and for the love that she has discovered that absolutely fills her to her brim. I am so thankful that she left, not because I don't love her deeply, but because I am proud of my best friend standing up for herself, even if that meant leaving. That must've been really hard for her. Love is not possession; she was never mine to keep in the first place. You must always give everybody back at some point, and none of it is in your control as much as you think that it is. Your parents, your children, your "best friends," your leaders - they are all temporary mirrors for each season of your life, some longer than others. That is why we must have ultimate gratitude for those who are fair to us, those who love us unconditionally and faithfully, those who are there for us in the dark corners that nobody else sees, and for those who stay to love us, even still. That is why we must draw very definitive boundaries for all else, so that they do not pull love from those who deserve to receive it from us the most. Relationships transitioning in your life are only life-shattering, catastrophic events if your ego is stronger than your faith. If you think that your plan was what was "supposed" to happen and you throw a fit for years when it doesn't go according to *your* plan, that's your ego thinking it has more control than the Universe around you, and that is one quick way to trap yourself in a hamster wheel of sadness and disappointment in this life.

None of this is in your hands.

Only your list of beliefs and how you choose to stand up for them consistently and endlessly.

CHAPTER 4: TAKING CARE OF YOUR SHELL

There are many practical ways for you to sharpen yourself and your tools for battle, as different as all our battles may be, our ways of preparation are all basically the same.

Your soul's mode of transportation in this lifetime happens to be the human being reading this. Regardless of how you *feel* about your body, the *fact* is, your body has been the only single thing there for you 100% of your life. It has protected you and shielded you and taken yours and others harm and abuse, all while healing itself and still waking you up each morning to a new opportunity for another day to try and be better than you were yesterday. It has been forgiving and pushed limits it didn't have to for you. It has respected your relationship with your mind and soul while you haven't. When will it be time for you to start showing your human shell gratitude for what it *is* for you, rather than picking it apart for what it *isn't*? When will your respect for your own body and long-term health be more important to you than your deceptive, short-term gratifications? Is getting healthy and re-training your body to do things it may have not done since you were a child hard? You're damn right, it is. But isn't it also hard being out of shape and not in balance with your health, suffering from all the disadvantages of what it steals from your everyday life, let alone your long-term life? It's challenging to consistently be physically active when you don't *feel* like being active, but it's much more sensible to endure that challenge and be gaining strength and mobility over time, rather than dealing with the hardship of being on the opposite trend of consistently feeling worse. There are practical ways to sharpen your human to function and *feel* better than you have ever felt in your life! Whether you need to lose body fat, gain lean mass, or just *feel* better and have more energy and a better overall health, I have found that there is basically one way every single person can start making progress using the same plan, just modifying it based on their goals.

As I had brought up earlier, like it or not, we have a relationship with every part of our existence. Your relationship between your soul and your physical human body is one of the most important relationships you will ever have the responsibility of taking care of, a lot of us just haven't been taught how. Have you ever been all gung-ho about beginning a new process of taking care of yourself and your mind and spirit are like, "Hell yeah, let's do it!"

But then your body is like, "Um, I don't know what the hell you think you're trying to do, but I do NOT think so!?"

Have you ever heard somebody say, "Your mind will take you places that your body doesn't even know it can reach!"

As far as your self-care, does it ever feel like you are in a constant, undefeatable battle within yourself, as if you had a demon on one shoulder and an angel on the other?

These are all very real and valid feelings and emotions you may be experiencing! It can feel defeating and hopeless at times. The most powerful tool I have given my clients and others that I love, is to begin treating your human body as your soul's child. It is your mind and soul's duty to lead your child/human body shell into health and consistency in providing great energy for your being. Most of us walk around allowing our childlike bodies to run our minds and souls and that is 100% backwards. Your body will respond to your thoughts, the same way as a child responds to its parents' lessons or demands. If your body (child shell) has been running the show for quite some time, then inevitably, you will deal with more resistance to new rules as you try to change your body's habits and routine. When your cravings come up, or your body is telling you that it just doesn't want to, it is vital to have a conversation from your soul to your body that things are changing, and this isn't the way the rules work within your household anymore. You must stand firm in your new boundaries, no matter how much your childlike shell tries to rebel against your authority. Take time to talk to your body, as if it were your innocent child that YOU led astray. Apologize for not taking better care of your body while you were lost or distracted in your process, thank your childlike shell for always being there for you and for being so forgiving for what you have put it through, and tell it that you will be investing more love and life into it than ever before, even when it gets tough.

Another relationship we share is with that in which we consume. I don't want you *feeling* like food is the enemy when food is a vital part of your existence. Food is not the bad guy, societal manipulation of foods for exposure or financial gains is the bad guy. A very large percentage of what is sold in grocery stores is more destructive for your health than productive. In places like Las Vegas, they manipulate the environment of the casinos, for their gamblers to be prone to spend more money; they make the floors busy, so it makes you dizzy to look at for too long-you must look up at what is around you. They enhance the oxygen in the buildings to make you breathe easier while you're there. They put winning slot machines on the aisle ends, so that oncoming tourists and passersby are tempted to try the machines too. You'll notice similar tactics in society with foods and beverages within advertising and within the stores themselves. Do you ever see commercials for vegetables and grass-fed meats and whole foods? Often, commercials and ads are to appeal to the children, who often are the ones determining what their parents will purchase for them. The kids are already in their parent's ears about their wants before they ever enter the front door of the store. Upon entrance to the store, right when you walk in, there are ads for items on sale all around you! The holiday candies and the chips and sodas on sale, etc. Then, around the perimeter of the store, separated from everything else, are your human's actual necessities - the fruits and vegetables, the meats and other produce, dairy and deli-fresh baked goods, etc. Most everything in the middle of the perimeter of the store is purposeless, a lot of it being more destructive for you than productive. EVERYTHING you consume is either productive, or destructive... there is no in-between. Before you consume it, you must ask what its *purpose* is. Six days of the week, your *purpose* of consumption should be strictly for energy, strength and function; it should be your gift to your human shell for its gift to you, which is the very air that you breathe. If what you're about to consume isn't benefiting your health, then it's inevitably pulling you away from it. If when you break down "why" you're about to consume it and it has no nutritional value, then the *purpose* of the consumption is for your deceptive cravings and feelings, not for your long-term health, not to mention the finances you just wasted. Our focus is now long-term, we are focused on a lifestyle, not a quick, temporary crash diet fix; be patient with yourself as you learn and adapt.

After several weeks of eating according to your health, rather than your feelings, you will begin to crave the feeling of eating clean over the feeling of satisfying a temporary craving. It gets easier and preferable over time. As much as I believe strongly in eating clean consistently as a lifestyle, I also believe just as strongly in treating yo'self occasionally! It isn't what you do occasionally that determines your lifestyle, it's what you do consistently that does. I give my clients one "treat day" each week. It isn't a "cheat day," what in the hell are you cheating on? Food is delicious and you should indulge in foods that taste so good your eyes roll back. Treat yo'self! If you treat yourself a little bit each day of the week, then you spend a little bit of each day burning off food, instead of your body fat, whereas if you just save it for that one day of the week, you can eat whatever the hell your cute little heart desires and burn *all* of it off the next day and start fresh again. You following me? I know it's a lot, but you deserve to hear it and to have the opportunity to take the best care of yourself possible. Just in switching to eating more purposefully for six days of the week, you will see progressive results in your energy levels, your hormonal balance, your physical appearance, mood, sleep, focus, and countless other pieces of your being. It is imperative to your health to be consuming a lot of water, as well! Your goal should be one gallon per day. Put a ruler up to the side of a gallon water jug and divide it into six equal sections. Label each section starting with the time you wake up, then labeling each section for two hours later, making 12 total hours of water consumption. This will break up your daunting gallon goal into several smaller, more seemingly achievable goals for the day. Any cravings you're having throughout the day that don't benefit your *purpose* aren't going to benefit your health; save it for your treat day, because they also serve a *purpose* at the right time.

As humans, we have what is called a mind/gut connection. A simple example of this is when we get feelings of nerves or anxiety, we tend to get "butterflies" in our tummy - this is just a minor form of the mind/gut connection. This is also why it's so important to trust your gut, it's more than likely a signal from your mind that you haven't acknowledged yet. Another form of mind/gut connection is our thoughts about what we are consuming. An example of this to me would be the modern day "Placebo Effect," giving patients virtually "fake" medications and with the patient's simple *expectation* for the pill to do something, it's possible for the body's own chemistry to cause effects that the medication would have. As humans, if we fixate on a craving too much, and don't detach from that *feeling*, then our bodies automatically begin to store fat before we ever even consume what we're thinking about. The *purpose* of "treat days" isn't for your body's health, it is for your mind's. Write down the craving, know that you will get to it on treat day, and let it go. It's all about balance, my friends. This process isn't about depriving you of things you enjoy, it's about finding alternatives for your destructive habits, which are much more sustainable for your long-term health and beliefs.

Another *fact* about your human is that it needs to be active sometimes, whether you *feel* like it, or not. We were meant to rest, but we weren't meant to live in rest. Balance. I've also seen humans addicted to too much activity and have deprived themselves of much needed rest; neither is a sustainable, long-term way to live healthiest. You need activity and you need rest; both will feel much better when paired together. You don't have to be in the gym to do it or use equipment or put pressure on yourself to be at a certain ability; you must just get up and get active and do your best each day. Start where you are right *now*. You have every resource of training at your fingertips on your phone! Literally *Google* or *YouTube* exercises based on what your goals are and find something that works for you! Each week, challenge yourself a little bit more. One hour of exercise a day is literally 4% of your entire day and it effects the entire other 96%. Exercise isn't just for your body, it releases the same chemicals that they put in anti-depressants, it helps with memory and your sleep patterns, it boosts confidence, it changes breathing patterns for everyday life, it changes everything. You don't need motivation, that is a fleeting *feeling*; you need some self-respect! You need the understanding that regardless of how you *feel*, your human deserves for you to show up and support it like it has supported your mind and soul.

How is your rest?

Do you take time to slow down and just *be*?

Why not? What are you running from?

"I sleep most of my days away."

What are you hiding from?

"I'm an insomniac."

Are you? Or, are you simply lying next to the wrong person at night? Maybe you're just too overrun by your life for your mind to quiet down and let you sleep? Are you an insomniac, or do you just lack peace?

One of the most powerful weapons of intention I have been developing in my life is waking up an hour earlier than I used to. My daughter wakes up around 7:00 a.m., so I am always up by 6:00 a.m. As I said before, everything should be done with purpose; I don't wake up to wander around the apartment and stare around wishing I was back in bed. I awake and practice gratitude by thanking my Universe for blessing me with the ability to still inhale and exhale the breath of life this morning, despite the magnitude of the hardships that have come at me. I press the "start" button on the coffee that I prepared the night before. I read… or some mornings, I write, or listen to faithful music and close my eyes. It's just Universe check-in time to lock into your beliefs and your purpose before you're confronted with the outside world for the day. It may be challenging at first, but if you're serious about making shifts in your life to bring you peace and joy consistently, you will prioritize new tools like this because they will make you *feel* better.

Your life hasn't been near as hard on you as you've been on yourself. The damage they did to you doesn't touch the damage you've inflicted onto yourself. They may be at fault for hurting you, but *you* are at fault for allowing it to hurt you repeatedly. Start being good to yourself *now*, nobody else is going to do it for you. Let's bring it back to the basics and start taking care of our bodies, then see how our minds respond. How the outside world will treat you, will be directly proportionate to how you will treat yourself.

CHAPTER 5: BALANCE

If I was to ask you what "mental health" looked like to you, what would you say?

What about if I asked you what "success" looked like to you?

For a lot of humans, "mental health" means happiness. And for a lot of humans, "success" means wealth.

You will never feel fully fulfilled or consistently joyous only acquiring finances. If you have the blessing, or curse, of showing up to your death bed, no amount of money will be there to hold your hand or extend love to you. No amount of money will keep your memory or example of God alive when you're gone. No amount of money will dab your dry lips or speak sweet, loving things to you during your final breaths. No amount of money will heal loneliness.

Only connections and relationships that were nurtured and tended to will be there. Only genuine love can bring you comfort and assurance of faith in where you're going. What matters here in this existence is truly immeasurable in price tags.

Just how wealth does not make you a success, happiness does not make you mentally healthy. This existence isn't all chalupas and pumpkin spice lattes, my friends, we are in a *living hell*! There are hard times and you won't always be happy. So, when you're feeling less than happy, does that make you mentally ill?

No, it makes you *human*.

There are moments of incredible triumph and happiness and celebration of life and love, there are moments of the deepest sorrow and pain you have ever felt, then there are all the moments in-between.

"There is an appointed time for everything.

And there is a time for every event under Heaven—

A time to give birth and a time to die; A time to plant and a time to up-root what has been planted.

A time to kill and a time to heal; A time to tear down and a time to build up.

A time to weep and a time to laugh; A time to mourn and a time to (laugh and) dance.

A time to throw stones and a time to gather stones; A time to embrace and a time to shun embracing.

A time to search and a time to give up as lost; A time to keep and a time to throw away.

A time to tear apart and a time to sew together; A time to be silent and a time to speak.

A time to love and a time to hate; A time for war and a time for peace."

-Ecclesiastes 3:1-8

It is mentally healthy to understand what you have control over and what you don't, to accept your feelings and soak in them, all the while knowing that they aren't *true,* and they don't define you. It is mentally healthy to be adaptable and to have a plan, but to also be willing to veer from it when you need to. It is mentally healthy to be able to constantly reflect on who you are and who you are becoming.

It is mentally healthy to have a balance in your life.

If you want to represent your God and the strength you have developed through your pain and be taken seriously in this life, **stand up straight.**

If you're leaning forward, you're living like a ticking time bomb, pissed off, stressed out and anxious, continually and defensively looking for what's coming next.

If you're leaning backwards, you're living in your heavy past, drowning in depression and regret. You have fallen victim to what was supposed to help you grow.

If you're leaning to the side, you are living for the acceptance and appeasement of others. You are living without a vision or purpose, just going through the motions of your stagnant waters. If you live a life to please others, that means you are willing to compromise your integrity and beliefs for somebody else's well-being above your own. It isn't your responsibility here to sacrifice your values for others' temporary well-being.

To attain balance is to stand up straight. To quote many others who have said it before me, *"Be where your feet are."* Be 100% present in every moment. If that in which is taking your time at that moment doesn't have a purpose for what life you dream of, you have the choice to leave it for something that will better serve you and your God. If you don't make the choice to stand up for where your time, love and energy is invested, then your life will inevitably find ways to pull you further from your goals. If what you're doing *does* reflect who you want to be, or *does* fill you up, then you owe it to that source of light to give it your undivided attention.

I had a woman come into the gym that I train at with her kids one day; one of our trainers had told her of a product she should invest in, so she was coming to investigate it and ask a couple of questions. Once we started digging into her life story a little bit, she said, "I just run 90 miles per hour ALL the time! I work out every day, but I must find ways to stay busy because I can't just work out all the time! I was up at 4:00 a.m. this morning on the treadmill because I couldn't sleep! My husband thinks I'm crazy!"

My soul immediately sank for her, as I understood all too well that it wasn't her body that couldn't calm down, it was her poor cute soul and brain. Her kids were looking up at us as we spoke and my heart broke for them, as I knew their mom must've been feeling this way for a lot of their lives, and they have been taught this standard of unhealthy business because their mom hadn't taken the time to slow down and confront her demons, in order to be more present for her kids.

I said to her, and if you are in her same position, I say to you, "My goodness, aren't you just waiting to collapse into safety? Your poor being needs *rest*. What are you running from? I can tell you right now it isn't a physical problem."

She became emotional and immediately broke, already knowing that how she has been living is unhealthy, just not knowing how to stop running.

My advice to her was to slow down. To be 100% present in each moment, so that she can decide if something brings her joy, or not. I told her not to focus on eliminating the dark because there is truly no such thing, but rather to focus on adding a little bit of light that's been missing each day until her days only consist of things that fuel her, instead of draining her. I told her, and I tell you, face yourself. Even if you don't like your reflection right now. Forgive yourself for who you haven't been and step into who you deserve to be.

If it's an issue of time management, sit down with a new daily planner and write what your "Ideal Schedule" would look like. Not what is happening now, but what kind of weekly schedule would bring you the most joy and allow you to be 100% present during each task. Then, make changes accordingly. You're allowed to have whatever schedule you would like, if it's helping your family grow. Every single section of your day in your planner should have something in it, even if it's relaxed YOU time. This will help you establish a more purposeful daily schedule of keeping productive, rather than staying in the hamster wheel cycle of busyness. If something comes up that isn't written in your schedule for the day, decide if it is more valuable for your overall purpose to veer from your schedule for the unplanned, or if it's a necessary time for you to stick to your schedule and say "No" to whatever human or task is asking for your attention. Saying "No" is not only okay, it's a powerful full sentence that you will need to use regularly, if you plan on being in control of your life!

When you spend time with your kids, be fully present and checked in to them. Listen to them and be bold enough as a parent and friend to ask them questions. They aren't yours forever, you must give them back to this big world one day and their relationship with you will then be up to *them.* Are you the kind of person they're going to want to be around as an adult when they finally do get to make a choice? Don't live a life that's so busy leaning forward, that you forget to invest your time and love into the souls and experiences that matter now; you will be busy preparing and planning for a future that never comes true. If you don't have children yet, please urge those that you love to invest time in theirs. Ask to hang out and do things with them *and* their kids. Loving them the best way is supporting where their focus should be and not selfishly getting mad when they need time with their kids, rather than go out and be irresponsible or distracted with you! They will gravitate towards your friendship and thank you one day when their kids are still their best friends as adults, too.

Start taking care of people who are good to you and show you continual love, before you go off searching for approval or acceptance or attention from humans you don't even know!

We all have our own versions of "cutting", some of them are just more apparent than others. Self-sabotage is slow suicide; whether it's picking at your skin until you bleed, eating your *feelings* away, running away from yourself as fast as you can, etc. We, as a collective, individually need to find ways to dig into our pain in ways that help us grow, rather than ways that kill us slowly. I used to punch walls as an angry child, so much so that the fibers of my skin fused to my knuckle bones. One of my teachers in high school once saw my hand and thought it was shattered and called my parents, whom I had hidden my hand from for weeks and my Dad had to take me to the hospital. After years of finding release or distraction in hitting things, I realized long-term that this wasn't doing anything but hurting myself physically AND emotionally and nothing on the inside of me was changing! There was no longer a purpose in doing it, other than getting occasional negative attention.

My sister introduced me to weightlifting. I started working out hard as hell, as she taught me proper form and technique. I would be at my gym multiple times a day some days during my hardest times of fighting my demons! I threw fucking fits inside of myself, screaming at my life with every rep! It hurt so bad sometimes, and still does when I'm having a battle kind of day. I can beat the living shit out of my entire body at the gym and when I walk out, I am **stronger,** and I am more in control and any of my less-than-great emotions or *feelings* are left on the floor when I leave! And check it out, no bloody knuckles to talk about, only muscles. You must learn to embrace your pain differently, more healthily, more sustainably. (I don't just mean through kicking your own ass in the gym, though I am an advocate of that.) Find something that doesn't distract you or help you run away from your demons, find something that forces you to confront them in a way that is healing, rather than destructive. Find a passion that lights you up! If you're struggling with finding your own, ask if there's any way you can help or join others with theirs! Try some new things out, let go of the ones you didn't care for, dive into the ones that you love!

Your time here is so priceless and irreplaceable, invest it wisely. If it doesn't help in your process of reaching your goals, or bring you great joy, then don't invest your time or valuable efforts of love on it anymore. Your long-term peace is worth way more than dead-end habits and meaningless company.

YOU do not need to be saved. You have just never been taught how to access all that power and love inside of you to save yourself! Once you find *that,* you will realize that you were made in God's exact image and you *are* part made fully of *Him,* you are just scared.

The Father, the Son and the Holy Spirit. The Holy Spirit is alive in YOU!

You asked God to do something and He *did,* he created a YOU!

YOU have the power to change this whole damn place!!

But it all must start with what you're willing to uncomfortably grow inside of you.

JUST BE.

To whomever is finding themselves reading this script that was sent to me, to deliver to you:

I cannot express or reiterate to you with enough authority, or power, or conviction, that **YOU,** right now in this very moment, are plenty! You are growing, and that is so gorgeous! But it is also really, exceptionally beautiful that you are still here in this existence with us, that you have made it to this point, and you are *still* fighting, regardless of your trauma. I find it to be such an act of love for yourself that you crave to more than just survive, but that you want to thrive and build and lead yourself closer to your light.

I want for each of you to know that through your hard work and growth, you are not becoming something new, you are only coming back home to who you were always meant to be. This life is about rediscovering your roots and watering and healing those, so we don't feel so exhausted on the hamster wheel of trying to "fix" our symptoms. Whoever/Whatever Maker created you, that was the same Maker who created the deepest oceans and the tallest forests, the most vicious and hungry of creatures, and the most delicate of flowers; the light of the day and the dark of the night! Whoever/Whatever your Creator is, thought you were enough to be here long before you ever made a choice in your life. You were already *enough* then. This isn't about becoming somebody that is accepted or validated, you already were. The world around you just told you otherwise. This is about coming back to who you have always been, who the world took you away from. This is about taking control of your life back and having so much genuine love for your own existence, that you can't help but pour it out onto others. Regardless of how you *feel,* something much bigger than you said that *you* belong here, no matter what any human has told or shown you otherwise. This isn't about you proving anything to anybody, this is about you going through this life feeling the best you possibly can, no matter what tries to come against you!

For a lot of us that are hard on ourselves, or constantly hungry for more, it can be difficult to feel like you are ever quite "enough". It is imperative that you take time to create a life that you desire through your actions and your determination and discipline, but also take time to soak in the present moment of gratitude and appreciation for your ability to even have the thoughts it requires you to get where you dream of going. Take time to soak in the fact that you are a complete and total badass already. The decisions you make through your days, routines and habits will either magnify your "badassness," or they will make you less of a badass. I suppose that's how you could summarize this entire book, just in that last sentence.

When your mind starts racing and you are now aware that your thoughts are not always (and are rarely) your *truth,* you can stand against those racing thoughts and literally say in a moment, "STOP." You have power over your thoughts. You can freeze your own state of mind and take as much time as you need to look at your situation from a birds-eye perspective. You can then decide, in a practical way, what the best solution is for whatever has come against your peace. When something out of your control presents itself to your path, take a moment to reflect on why you are affected before you react. Respect your past traumas by taking them into account. Respect your established boundaries because of your past lessons, before you react or make decisions based on past impulsive responses that leave you in a cycle of dependency or the same repeated mistakes (decisions).

With your shift of focus and perspective of *why* things have happened for you in your life, rather than happening *to* you, you will find a deeper purpose in even just breathing the air that you breathe. That will unlock daily joy in the process, rather than only in temporary highs of reaching milestones. Once you reveal this for yourself in your own existence, it is vital to share that reached level of love with those around you, even if they don't "deserve" it. Love doesn't always make sense; that's what makes it so much fun! It defies reason and facts and odds; it is relentless in its pursuit; it doesn't care what rules or judgement tries to hold it back; it will always prevail. Love always wins. Choose to love this life you're living right now, and anything that is getting in the way of that, change it. Don't accept a life that isn't yours to live. There is so much more out here waiting for you, and it has only *your* name on it. You are built up of what it will take to get to it, you just have to reveal that power to yourself through acting on love and gratitude *right now* and trusting that your God/Universe will guide your steps, once you decide to stand up and put one foot in front of the other.

You are worthy.

You are valuable.

You are strong.

You are courageous.

You are built of your own magic.

You are enough.

We can do better.

Let's keep planting our seeds; our harvest will catch up to us!

I love you.

What I've Been Taught	What I Believe

www.ingramcontent.com/pod-product-compliance
Lightning Source LLC
Chambersburg PA
CBHW051122250726
48655CB00007B/2832